In His Heart

Written by Aub

Copyright © 2024 by Aubrey Clarke
All rights reserved. No part of this book may be reproduced, stored in a retrieval system, or transmitted in any form or by any means, electronic, mechanical, photocopying, recording, or otherwise, without the prior written permission of the author, except in the case of brief quotations embodied in critical articles and reviews.
This is a work of fiction. Names, characters, businesses, places, events, and incidents are either the products of the author's imagination or used in a fictitious manner. Any resemblance to actual persons, living or dead, or actual events is purely coincidental.

Published by Envision Urban
ISBN: 978-1-988785-12-7
For permissions requests, write to the publisher at:
info@envisionurban.com

First Edition

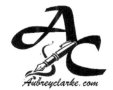

About The Author

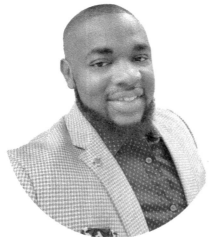

Aubrey Clarke is an inspiring author, poet, spoken word artist and storyteller.
Born in Guyana South America and immigrated to Canada as a young child. He has released several children's books and is a preferred speaker at many organizations. He is a Media Sales and Marketing Professional as well as an event promoter. He loves leaving a positive change in the lives of everyone he comes in contact with. He is extremely proud that his timeless work will live on for centuries after he is gone.

A Word From the Author

This book is a compilation of poems that I've composed over the years, drawing from both my own experiences and the perspectives of others. These words are meant to evoke a range of emotions and may remind you of moments you've lived through.

I hope this work helps you find the strength to forgive yourself and others, allowing you to move forward and become the best version of yourself.

My deepest desire is that these poems inspire and motivate you to love yourself and others in a healthy, meaningful way.

CONTENTS

Baby Give Me A Chance...7
A Vision...8
I Love You..9
The Melody In My Heart..10
As The Flower Blossoms...11
Loving You Until The End Of Time.................................12
Angel Eyes..13
If I Could Grow Wings..14
When It's Not Shared With You....................................15
Before You Go..16
Beauty Is What You Are...17
Burning Flame..19
Is It Really You..20
Surrender...21
The Flower Before Your Eyes......................................22
The Autumn Leaves...23
Virtuous Woman..24
Share With Me..26
I Must Be A Fool...27
Please Be Gentle..29
I Stand Amazed..30
As Fast As Lightning Flashes.....................................31
A Portrait Of Love...32
If You Only Knew...33
If I Ever Had A Wish...35
Deep Inside...36
There's Something About You.....................................37
Conceptual Prayer...38

You Are Worthy..39
My 2-Lip..41
The Thief...42
He Cries..43
Do You Understand..45
I Can Never Forget..46
You Said You'd Never Leave..48
The Fall..50
What Am I Doing Here..52
A Moment Gone..54
The Sun Has Come Out..55
You Escalated...56
The Time Has Come..57
To Miss You...58
Candy Love...59
Loving You Without A Reason..60
When I Love Again..61
Sealed, Unsealed, Sealed...62
The Journey Is Over..63

IN HIS HEART

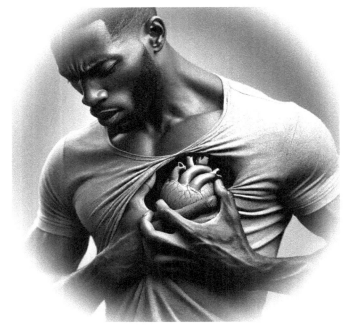

by Aubrey Clarke

His heart is strong, yet delicate.
His heart is fierce, yet intricate.
Be his place of safety so that he can protect you.
Every man longs for the one he can treasure forever.
As you read this book, think about whether you are helping him heal or breaking him down.
Men, as you read this, examine yourself so that you can be the best version of yourself and love healthily.

{A Vision}

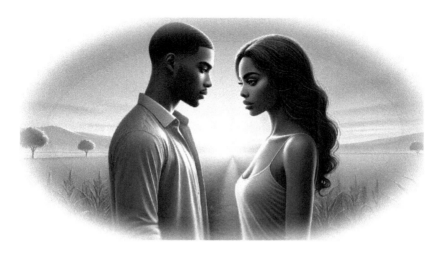

When I look into your eyes, I begin to see the completion of my vision.
I see purpose in you. I see a life full of memories, full of joy, full of love, and determination.

For I am in pursuit of purpose
and as my life begins to unfold
before my eyes, I see you in the center of the fold.

The Word says, "The two shall become one," and as I see you in my vision,
I see me.

{Baby Give Me A Chance}

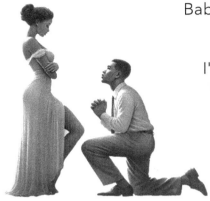

Baby, give me a chance.
Don't close the door
on romance.
I'm a man of integrity.
I'm a man who wants
you next to me.

I'm mesmerized
by your radiance.
I am captivated
by your brilliance.
I can't put up a resistance,
especially in your presence.
Absent, or face to face,
I long to be wrapped
in your embrace.
When you draw me
into your realm,
I am overwhelmed.

Baby, don't let this opportunity pass us by.
Don't let this precious moment die.
Nobody knows what will be tomorrow.
But be sure that I'll gladly bear your sorrow.
So come now, and let us reason together,
and I'll pledge to love you forever.
Come fly with me on eagle's wings.
Let me be your king.
You've thrown me into a passionate trance.

So baby, please, give me a chance.

{I Love You}

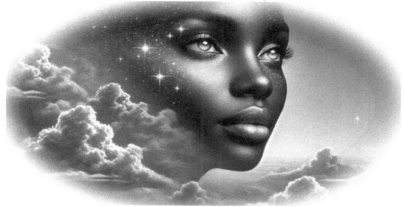

I love you, yes, I do
and my love for you is true.
More than I can show,
more than you could ever know.

If you searched every section of my heart,
you'd find your name,
and if I searched yours, I hope it would be the same.

If all the stars were missing from the sky,
I would still have two in your beautiful eyes.
You are like the rainbow after the rain,
and your smile eases my deepest pain.

If you were a book and I could read you, the only
words that I would see,
would be the sentence saying you are extreme beauty.
Without a doubt I can say,
that you are the expression of sweetness in every way.

{The Melody In My Heart}

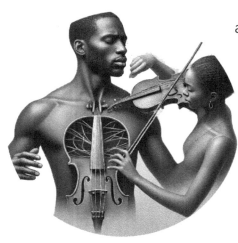

My heart is a violin,
and you are the bow,
together we make
beautiful
music you know.

If my heart
had a million locks,
you would hold the
key to every door,
and I would love
you more and
more and more.

You are the flower and I am the bee,
when you put us together it's instant honey.
It's true, we were meant to be.
The Lord has brought us together, it's our destiny.
What a joy it is to look upon your face.
Thank God, that you're an expression of His grace.

Happy times will come and happy times will go,
I am so thankful that
through it all our love will grow.
If you were a book and I could read you, the only
words that I would see,
would be the ones saying you are extreme beauty.
Without a doubt I can say,
that you are the expression of sweetness in every way.
There is forever in my heart a melody,
singing, my precious we were meant to be.

{As The Flower Blossoms}

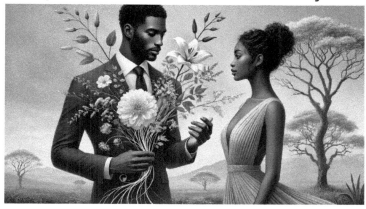

As the flower blossoms when spring draws near,
my heart blossoms for you my dear.
As its aroma fills the summer breeze from north to south and east to west,
so too, your fragrance to me is the best.

The beauty of the flower is so very rare,
just as your beauty is beyond compare.
For the Lord is the creator of all below and all above,
so He created you a precious dove.

As the rain comes to make the flower grow,
you're the sun that melts the snow.
The glory of the stars in the sky,
can't compare to your beautiful eyes.

You are the sweetness of God's perfection,
in your face is his gracious reflection.
As the flower blossoms when spring draws near,
my heart blossoms for you my dear!

{Loving You Until The End Of Time}

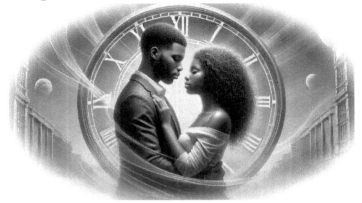

My love, I'll hold you in my arms,
and let you feel my charm.
I'll cherish and protect you.
Honey, you're one person I'll never neglect,
it's true.

I'll tell you that I love you in every way,
then I'll prove it to you by showing you every day.
I'll sing you sweet melodies all night long.
My baby, I'll never do you wrong.
I'll let the whole world know you're mine,
while I'm loving you until the end of time.

Admiring the radiance of your beauty, the glittering of
your eyes, the heart-heating sound of your voice and
your smooth, soft skin.
But I'm treasuring most of all what lies within.

My heart is playing the most romantic chimes.
Darling, while I'm loving you,
loving you until the end of time.

{Angel Eyes}

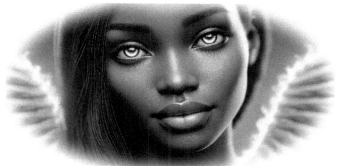

Angel Eyes is what I call you,
cause you inspire me to grow wings and fly.
Who needs drugs when you make me feel so high?

If the eyes are the window to the soul, then I see heaven inside of you.
I see a woman searching for someone who will be true.
Your personality is miraculous.
Lady love, you leave me feeling so gracious.
Your eyes are like a remote control; with each blink,
I sink a little deeper into you.

You speak with such compassion and love,
my treasure from above.
Give me your hand, and I'll never let it go.
Give me your heart, and I'll safeguard it forever.
Give me your body and I'll respect it with pleasure.
Give me your friendship and your ship will never sink.
All you have to do, Angel Eyes, is look at me and blink.

{If I Could Grow Wings}

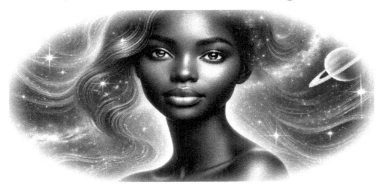

If I could grow wings, I'd fly you way up high.
so that you could be the prettiest star in the sky.
If I could grow wings, I'd take you to travel the solar system,
so that the whole galaxy could glisten, sparkling with our love.

If I could grow wings, I'd take you to sit in the clouds as the breeze would blow,
and I'd watch your spirit flow.
The entire sky would then glow, with the radiance of your beauty.

Yes, if I could grow wings we'd go up
and never come down,
forever filled with happiness, no more to frown.

If I could grow wings, I'd paint a rainbow of our love in the sky,
a covenant of promise sealed before our eyes.
If I could grow wings, I'd fly you way up high,
so that you could be the prettiest star in the sky.

{When It's Not Shared With You}

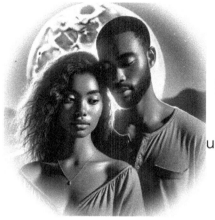

What is a smile when
it's not shared with you?
What is money and
priceless fortunes without
a love that's true?
What is a walk
underneath the moonlight,
when you're not
there to hold me tight?

What is a breath of fresh air,
my love, when you're no longer here?
I'm missing you with everything in me.
Now I'm here alone to face the stormy sea.

With waves of turmoil, lightning of loneliness,
and thunders of emptiness raging in my heart,
remembering when you did depart.

How could I leave my first love?
What was I thinking of?
Why did I leave your hands?
Why didn't I understand
that you were shaping me,
into what I needed to be?

I've learned a lesson so true,
finding out what life is like when it's not shared with
you.

{Before You Go}

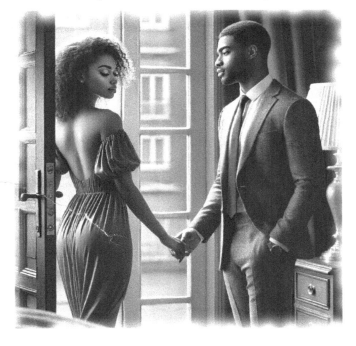

Before you go, there is something I'd like to say.

Before you go, there are memories I'd like to make.

Before you go, there are special moments I'd like to share.

Before you go, there's something I'd like to happen.

Before you go, there's something I'd like to do.
I want to look you in your eyes and say, I love you!

{Beauty Is What You Are}

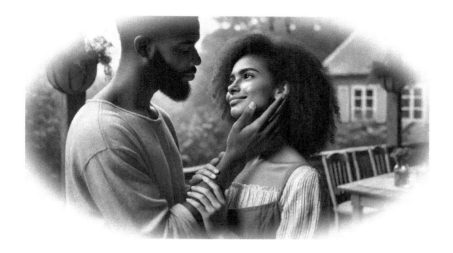

Beauty is what you are;
there is no comparison.
I searched near and far.

I searched the diamond mines of Africa, and the
precious stones there just couldn't do,
I searched the Egyptian pyramids, and the bounties
there couldn't compare to you.

I searched the meadows and hidden valleys.
I picked rare flowers, roses, and lilies.
I dove the deepest seas.
I climbed the highest mountains.
I visited the Aztec ruins.
I went to the Amazon jungle.
I became desperate

and searched every
antique collection, and art gallery,
I saw the Mona Lisa.
I even examined the Queen's treasures,
and there wasn't one that could measure,
up to your beauty.

I envisioned you walking across the constellations and
the whole universe stood still in awe
because of your magnificence.

One thing is for sure,
you were created in God's image and you are the one
my heart adores.
Beauty is what you are.
I searched near and far.
There was none that could compare.
For beauty, beauty, beauty is what you are!

{Burning Flame}

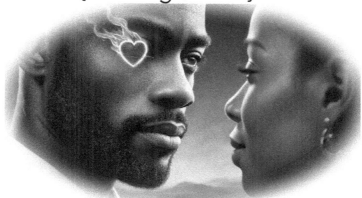

There is a burning flame in my eyes as I look upon you.
Can it be quenched?
Never, as long as you continue to amaze me with your overwhelming presence.

The flame begins to grow brighter each time you are in my presence,
causing my whole being to feel lighter,
until I am drawn out of my body,
floating in my subconscious, being guided by the irresistible aroma of your allure,
longing to be joined with the source of that sweet savour.

My eyes are now burning with love,
until my heart has now caught on fire.
You have become an intimate part of my desire,
for you are now one with the flame!

{Is It Really You}

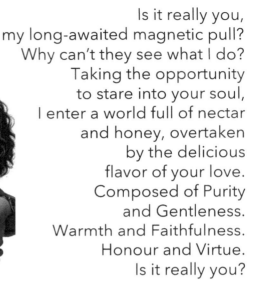

Is it really you,
my long-awaited magnetic pull?
Why can't they see what I do?
Taking the opportunity
to stare into your soul,
I enter a world full of nectar
and honey, overtaken
by the delicious
flavor of your love.
Composed of Purity
and Gentleness.
Warmth and Faithfulness.
Honour and Virtue.
Is it really you?

Floating in the place where my heart sings softly on a
stream made of syrup,
joined in harmony with the Source
and Essence of this land.

As I retract from this world of euphoria, I behold a
magnificent sight, which the radiance of the sunrise
and splendor of the sunset could not compare to.
For your overwhelming beauty has drawn me back
into the land of ecstasy, to taste of the chocolate-
covered candy of your love.

Is it really you, my sugarcoated destiny?
Is it really you, my long-awaited wife-to-be?
Is it really you?

{Surrender}

Surrender! With you I stand!
Confused?
Sister, I am a real man willing
to hold your hand.
In the solitude of your heart, I shall become a
part of your desires.
I am going to set your soul on fire.

I shall ignite you with all
my might and virtue. When you feel my passion
so warm and tender, baby, surrender!
You'll glow when you feel my tranquil flow,
of soft caress as I stroke your,
mind and relieve your stress.

There'll be no uncertainty
when I take you on a journey of ecstasy,
you next to me, my arms of power will be your
security! You transcend the boundaries of beauty
taking loveliness to another level where no woman has
gone before. You fill my eyes with splendor.

Your body that has more curves than a roller coaster
causes my blood vessels to boil and my heart to beat.
So, I've arrived at this conclusion that we need to start
a fusion, with all this heat!

I know for the time being I may be something of an
enigma but when you denude who I really am and you
feel my embrace so soft and my lips so tender,

Baby, I know you'll surrender!

{The Flower Before Your Eyes}

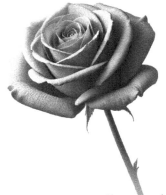

The pain you feel
inside won't last forever.
Like this precious rose,
both beauty and
thorns grow together.
To make the flower grow,
it takes the sun and the rain.
Just like you grow when
you face both joy and pain.
It will soon be over the rainbow will come out.
It will soon be over things will be turned about.

Outside, you're smiling.
Inside, you feel like you're slowly dying.
"When will this all end?" is what you often say.
You can no longer pretend that everything is okay.
Not even the rain can stop the rose from blossoming.
Not even the pain can stop you from shining.
Trials are nothing but stepping stones.
You are never alone.

So don't give up on your dreams.
If flowers were royalty, you'd be the Queen.
For your beauty, your elegance flows out of your essence.
Like the rose bringing to my nose, the sweetest fragrance.

Whenever you encounter problems, despite the size,
remember this precious flower before your eyes.

{The Autumn Leaves}

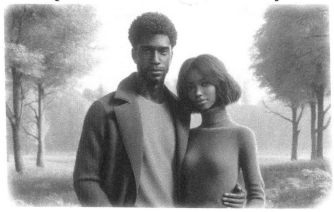

I see the leaves blowing in the breeze.
Autumn is here, and so many beautiful colours surround me.
The great waters, trees, and the animals—
nature working in harmony.

The sun, the moon and the sky so blue;
this world was made for me and you.
But there are no colours in my world.
If you're not beside me, girl.
Red and yellow.
Black and white.
Green, purple, brown, and blue—
you're the rainbow in my life.

Girl, I love you.
You've become my inspiration.
Come share in my salvation.
Let the autumn colours be
an example of the joy you bring me

{Virtuous Woman}

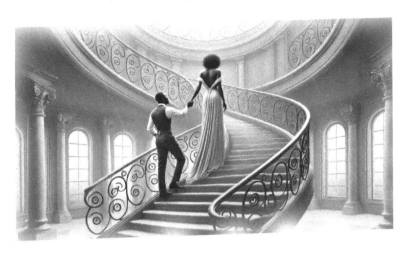

many men have walked out and left their children
and women alone.
once compassionate, tender heart of flesh has
become a raging fortress of stone.

iad of women are singing that sad song,
, oh where have all the good men gone?"
eel that you're at the end of your
t Virtuous woman, there is hope.
God comes into a man's heart,
's when true love starts.
vill stay and never depart.
at I will never leave you alone.

oman, I stand in awe of your
of your loveliness.
and I pledge to you, my
ness.

For so long, you've been used and abused,
but I refuse to confuse your mind,
cause you're my priceless treasure to find.
I recognize that you were oppressed,
and you fought to survive with that great strength that you possess.
Cover me, please with the prayers of thy security.
Cause me to shine with the radiance of true love,
which comes from above.
There is no other woman that I desire to climb with me up higher.

Stand by my side, always abide.
Virtuous woman, I've come to understand that
I need you to hold my hand.
I need you just as much as you need me.
Go with me to a place called heaven
and share my destiny.

As a circle has no beginning and no end,
you were meant to be my eternal friend.
Sweet lady, you cause my heart to sing.
I need you my Virtuous Queen
and I know you deserve a King.

So, let's not waver from left to right.
Walk with me straight ahead on that righteous path
and share my light,

Cause Virtuous woman, you're part of my heart's delight.
So please let it be known,
that I will never leave you alone.

{Share With Me}

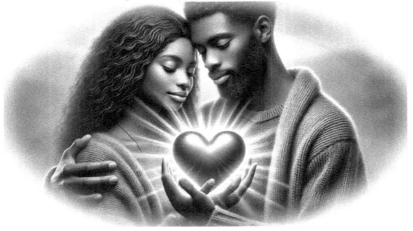

Share with me all of your concerns.
For you to be joyful, my heart doth yearn.

Share with me your memories, whether bad or good
and when you're finished sharing, you'll know I've understood.

Share with me today, and I'll stay until tomorrow.
Share with me your life so I can pray away your sorrows.

Share with me your love, share it so sweetly.
And I'll give you my whole heart,
I'll give it completely.
Don't be afraid of the way I make you feel.
Fantasies leave beautiful memories, but this one is for real.
Share with me.

{I Must Be A Fool}

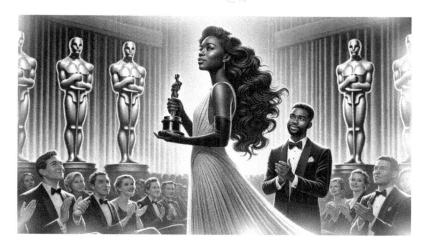

I must be a fool to ever think that I'll have you.
But if being a fool is what I have to be to let hope survive,

then a fool is what I am to keep my love for you alive.

How can I move when my heart beats to your groove?

When you speak, my heart stands at attention, awaiting your command.
I close my eyes and enter another dimension, and there we are standing hand in hand.

I've drunk of your potion.
I'm sinking in your ocean.
I don't mind drowning here for I've reached my promised land flowing with milk and honey, more irreplaceable than jewels and money.

I must be a fool to think that in the mornings when my eyes open, we'll actually meet lip to lip and be in each other's grip, while I slowly suck those fingertips.

A fool to think that I'll have that precious hair all over my face as I press my hard pecs against you in a warm embrace.

Fool, fool, fool to imagine that I'll ever lay with you beside a cozy fireplace, cuddling and talking all night long as the radio plays our favourite song.

A fool to think that I'll lay you down in a warm tropical place as I feed you your most desired food and you savour the taste.

A fool to think I'll be there with you when you win your first Academy Award and Grammy.

A fool to think that I'll be there in the hospital room when you start your own family.

But if being a fool is what I have to be to let hope survive,

then a fool is what I am to keep my love for you alive.

{Please Be Gentle}

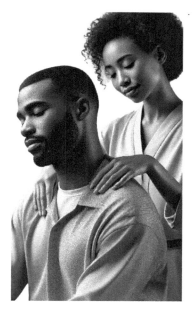

Please be gentle with me.
I'm like a delicate flower
that must be handled
with care.
Please shower me with
your love and draw near.

Don't feed me too much,
I will swell up and die.
Don't apply too much heat,
the bed that I lay
in will dry out.
Nourish me with sincerity,
faithfulness,
and understanding.
When the storms come,
I will be left standing.

Open up to me and rub me
softly with who you really are.
Stroke me with the gentle caress of
mental stimulation instead of erotic sensations.
Join your heart with mine in unity, never allowing
perplexity.

The harmony of our spirits in God will make sure that
we never become frauds.
This might sound sentimental, but baby,

please be gentle!

{I Stand Amazed}

How can it possibly be true,
that God would have
made perfection
when He created you?
That He would make your
smooth brown skin
out of milk chocolate.
That your hair would
flow like a gentle stream.
That your aura would
dictate you a queen.

Your elegance
leaves me fazed,
I stand amazed.
As your personality captures me,
your beautiful eyes hypnotize.
How can there be any resistance to your lovely
fragrance?
You are like a flower in full bloom, adding beauty to
any room.
So talented.
So fine.
So sweet.
So complete.

To describe you, there really is no phrase.
So, soft and tender lady, I stand amazed!

{As Fast As Lightning Flashes}

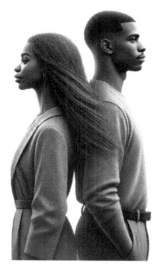

As fast as lightning
Flashes, life changes.
Like a Shakespeare drama,
life has so many stages.
Understand, maybe?
Overstand, baby?

Life is pain. Life is joy.
Life is you. Life is me.
Life is not guaranteed.
Today you're here.
Tomorrow you're gone.
Life feels too much to bear.
But somehow, I keep strong.

Life is not yesterday,
nor is life tomorrow.
Life is now; choose joy over sorrow.
Life is death and death is life.
To live, you've got to kill a lot of
the pain that's held you back.
To die is to be born again.
Just like a seed begins to grow after the rain.
Life is what you make it. Can you shape it?

Life is trust and honesty. Life is you and life is me.
Life is inside of the Almighty.
As fast as lightning flashes, life changes.
I pray that we'll never end up
being strangers, in life.

{A Portrait Of Love}

If I could paint a
portrait across the sky,
I'd paint a picture of
you so I could always
stare into your beautiful eyes.
And as the day turned to night,
like the stars, your eyes
would shine so bright, and I would envision holding
you tight, until dawn's early light.

If your eyes would ever close,
I'd paint a picture of a rose
and paint your smile to light the night,
then my heart would ignite, and I would love you with
all my might.
If your eyes opened again,
tears of joy would remove my pain.

Just to make this vision a reality,
I'd paint a picture of you and me.
Then I'd give you that painted rose,
around you my arms would gently close.
The stars would dim to set the mood.
The Milky Way would begin to flow,
the clouds would form our bed and pillow.
The Big Dipper formed the hot tub.
The Little Dipper, the oil to rub as our lips came
together, it was lightning and thunder.
Ring, ring, I did awake.

I guess I'll have to wait till next time to paint the church
bells and wedding cake.

{If You Only Knew}

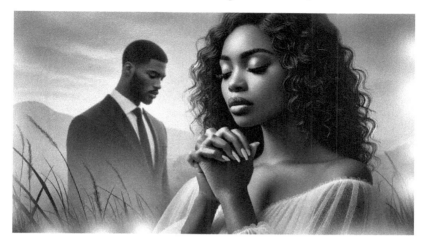

If you only knew, if you could only see, how happy we could be.
If you could just have one taste of my chocolate passion, oozing with flavor, for you to savour.

Throw your arms around me and feel my hot, steaming chest against your warm, succulent breast.

Feel my electric lips while you're still in my grip, let us lock at the hips.
Blaze me with the fire beaming in your eyes.
Comfort me with the warmth rising from your thighs.

But most of all, speak to me with your soft, paralyzing voice.
Stimulate me with your brilliance.
Energize my spirit and my soul.
Pray for my salvation and make me whole.

Electrify the very essence of my being.
Call me your lord, baby, and I'll call you,
my queen.

Now that you're at the point of gratification,
let me take you beyond the point of satisfaction.
Cause you have never reached your climax
until you've been with your destiny, that's a fact.
First, we'll get married and you'll wear my ring,
and your heart will sing like the songbirds in the spring.

Now, where should I start, from your toe to your head,
or from your head to your toe.
It doesn't matter because I promise you like a river any which way you will flow.

Do you think you can keep your poise without making too much noise?
For I'm about to flip you from side to side and all around.
I'll make you so high you aren't ever coming down.
Yes, wifey, if you only knew,

If you could only see, how happy we could be!

{If I Ever Had A Wish}

If I ever had a wish, I'd give my wish to you,
so that all your dreams, girl, would always come true.

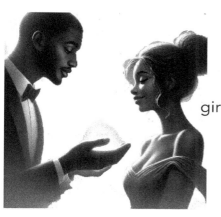

If I got a second wish,
I'd wish your wish was me,
so you and I, baby,
could be a happy family.
I would love you forever,
girl, and make you my world.
Just say you'll share my
Universe, and we'll be
walking hand in hand.
Together we will stand,
we will stand.

If I could paint a perfect sky I'd paint a canvas of you.
Your smile would be the sun
and the sky would be so blue.

If anyone was crying, I'd tell them to look up.
If anyone was dying, I'd say don't give up.
Cause you bring hope to hurting world, for man,
woman, boy and girl.
You're someone who understands,
a vital part of God's plan,

So, if I ever had one wish, if I could paint a perfect sky,
it would speak about how much I love you,
tell about how you make me fly.

{Deep Inside}

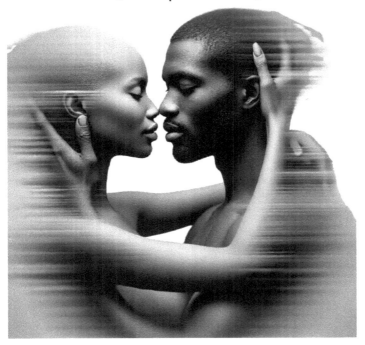

Deep inside your eyes there's a lioness waiting to roar.
Deep in your heart, there's a kitten waiting to purr.

Deep in your mind, there are fantasies
waiting to be lived.
Deep inside me, there's something
special I'm waiting to give.

You can be my roadmap and lead
me to your buried treasure.
I can be your King and cherish you forever.

Walk deep inside of me, and I'll walk deep inside of
you, and make your every wish and dream come true.

{There's Something About You}

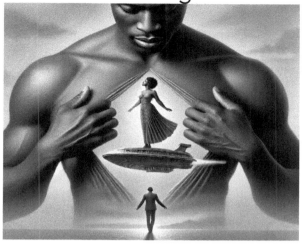

There's something about you that intrigues me.
There's something about you that fascinates me.
There's something about you that makes me dream of
cozy fireplaces and quiet streams.

Like the Starship Enterprise, you've gone where no
woman has gone before,
igniting the fire in my eyes as my passion
burns once more.
My hope has been restored, and I feel assured.

Let this moment be to you everything, girl,
you wished could be true.
Feel the power of my emotion.
Drink from my love potion.
Swim with me through life's ocean.
Taste my devotion.

Sugar, you make me feel brand new.
There's just something about you.

{Conceptual Prayer}

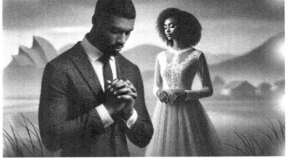

I prayed to God and asked Him to
send the perfect girl.
Then you came and changed my world.
You descended from a celestial place to ascend in my
heart. Your words kissed my soul.
Your gaze turned on my passion like a remote control.

I am enraptured by you.
Let us forge a kingdom together.
Let us merge our hearts forever.
You are to me everything that a woman could be.
You are to me everything that a friend should be.
Miraculously, I am taken to euphoric heights as your
touch plays my cells like a symphony
in perfect harmony.
Yes, there is music in your fingertips and comfort in
your lips.

You have rekindled my capacity to dream, and I aspire
to be the protector, the provider that you longed for,
all that you need and more.
I am so glad that you believed.
For, in my prayers, you were conceived.

{You Are Worthy}

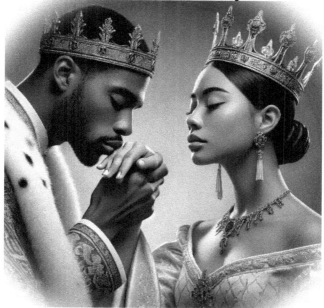

Hola, my queen, I know you're afraid to unlock the gates to the citadel that guards your being.
The secrets you conceal are covered with barbed wire.
Bringing them to the surface feels like you are going to set your life on fire.

The shame and the pain forced on you
by those who stole your choice.
I'll be here to help you find your voice.
Battling the silent thoughts that yell, it's all your fault.
Instead of living free, you lock yourself deep in a vault.

Inside you are screaming, someone please rescue me from this nightmare.
Then you turn to denial, sabotaging every relationship because of fear.

Counseling appears too terrifying because of what it may uncover.
But baby, you will discover, I want to help you heal, I'll be that lover.

Lay your head on my chest and let the beat of my heart speak words of affirmation into your soul.
Let me help you to regain control.
The emptiness that engulfs you from great loss will be filled.
I am just so thrilled to say, you are worthy.
Worthy to be made whole again.
Worthy to release the pain.

I will stand with you.
Stand in front of every force that tries to bring you back to a dark place.
Because together there isn't anything we cannot face.

So, exhale, and let us run the trail, called abundant life, my muse, my future wife.

{My 2 - Lip}

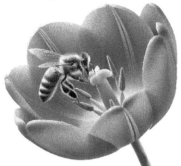

Spring is here, causing me to think of you once again.
I visualize you as a beautiful tulip in full blossom, and me as a bee gently crawling up the stem, causing the tulip to bend back and forth and side to side.

When the bee finally reaches the fruit, which is the blossom, it smoothly makes its way between the petals of the tulip into its center
sucking its sweet, luscious nectar.

Then it softly brushes against the tulip's stigma, causing it to clench.
At that same time, the sun radiates its intense heat down onto the tulip and the bee, energizing them for a few minutes which seems like an eternity.

In passion, the bee slides its way back down the stem causing the tulip to bend back and forth
and side to side.

The tulip then closes in satisfaction
as the bee buzzes in ecstasy.

{The Thief}

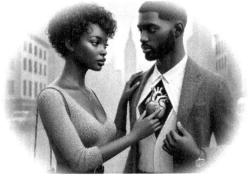

She crept oh so softly.
She moved oh so gently.
She smiled oh so sweetly.
Her words were the rhythm that
my heart danced to.
Her touch sent fuel through my being
Her lips ignited the flame that still burns with vigor.
When I was in her embrace,
there wasn't a problem I could not face.

One silent night, she crept out, oh so softly.
When the door to my chest shut, I awoke,
to find that she left with my heart—was this a joke?
But reality set in when, night after night, I heard the
hollowness of my empty chest echoing in the dark.
Oh, for my love to return and reignite the spark,
so that blood can once again
flow through my veins, fill this void, and remove the
pain.

For what is a man without his heart?
What is love at first sight,
when friendship ends before it ever starts?

{He Cries}

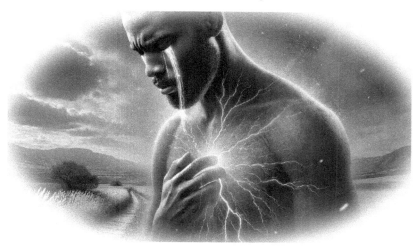

He cries, but the tears drip down the inside of his eyes to his soul while you perceive that he has no feelings. He cries but holds it deep inside as his pride and society tell him that a man's tears make him weak.

He cries in bouts of anger because to express himself any other way may taint his name and add to the pain.
He cries in the arms of another woman, self-sabotaging himself in lustful bliss because the one at home doesn't understand him.
He cries in silence and withdraws his hugs and words of affirmation while an inner stream
of salt drips to his heart.

The constant nagging and complaining instead of kind expressions of restoration.
The selfish desires and demands, always taking, leaving him feeling empty instead of filling his being with the passion that once burned.

I hear you. Right now, you are saying, "What about the things he does to me?"
The reality is, only acts of love will set you both free from the frustration of this dysfunctional world.
Heal yourself and help him heal instead of tit for tat and pain for pain; there is no gain.

He cries, longing for the mother who abandoned him as a child.
He cries, longing for a relationship with the father he was told did not want him.

A man trapped, battling the isms and skims of society, yet when he comes home there is no peace.
He cries, and with each tear drop, a part of him dies.

Where is the love he was promised?
Where is the woman that inspired him to ask for her hand?
Where is the woman who can help dry his eyes?
The woman who made him feel like he had received his greatest prize.
Where is the one who will motivate him to seek healing whether it be through therapy or her warm embrace giving him a safe place?

He cries—can you hear it through his silence?

{Do You Understand}

Understand?
Can you comprehend, or do you pretend,
that you know the horrific feeling
that overshadows me?
Do you see my hurt when I smile?
Can you feel my pain when I laugh?

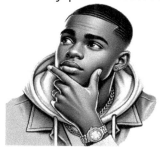

Do you understand?
Will you hold my hand and help me stand?
Of course not!
Have you forgotten that what you see on the outside
might be hiding what is on the inside.
In you, can I confide?
Will you abide, even when I've cried?
Will I know you've tried, or will I find out that you lied?

Can you see what I feel?
Can you relate to my agony?
Are you fooled by my apparent joy?
Do you know my reality?

Understand?
Will you hold my hand and help me stand?
Can you comprehend, or do you just pretend?

{I Can Never Forget}

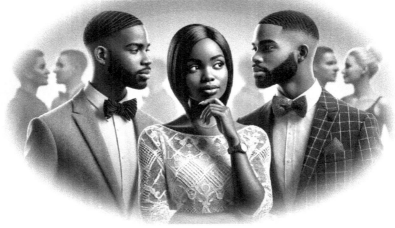

I can never forget the moment when you radiated in my presence and my eyes were entranced by you.

It was like you materialized from the celestial plane and caused me to believe in love again.
I can never forget the hope that filled my heart.
Could you be the one who has evaded me for so long?
Could you be my song?

I can never forget the way I felt
every time I saw your smile.
It's locked in my memory like a top-secret file.

I can never forget when I thought my dreams were fulfilled as we bonded over deep conversation.
It was good vibrations.

Your hug and your smell energized every cell.
I was as excited as kid at show and tell.

I can never forget when the fear of losing our friendship if things didn't work out caused you to choose another.
You made him your lover.
Yet I was your confidant,
the one you turned to for advice.
The one you called late at night.

Time passed, and you clashed.
Like a drunk driving fast, your relationship crashed.
You came back, but I could never forget.

I was broken, but I was strong.
I was hurt, mostly because I was wrong about you being my song.

I hold no grudge.
I still got love.

But I can never forget,
that you made the wrong bet.

{You Said You Would Never Leave}

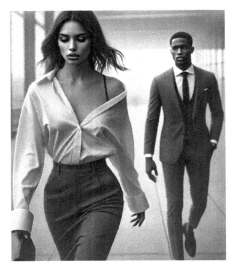

You said you would
never leave,
you promised you'd
always stay.
Just when I needed
you most,
you picked up and
threw me away.

Were promises meant
to be broken?
Were promises meant
to be kept?

When you broke yours, I surely wept.

You said we would be together,
always and forever.
You said you'd leave me never.
I cried when I realized that you lied.
Broken beyond repair, you never really cared,
I now know the memories were never shared.

Years gone to waste, leaving me a bitter taste.
Every joyful moment forgotten.
A relationship gone rotten.
How could this be? You never loved me.

God is Love.
His Love is enduring, long-suffering, patient and forgiving—that's not the kind you are living.

There is a saying that is so true, that what goes around comes around, and this saying also applies to you.

It is God's law that all must reap what they sow.
When your time comes you will surely, surely know!

You said you'd never leave,
you led me to believe!

{The Fall}

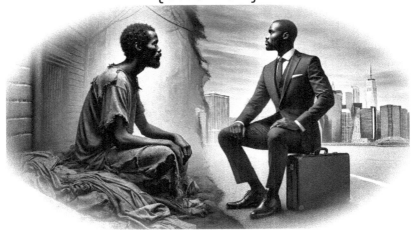

I had it all!
How did I fall?
I was a successful businessman
whom so many admired.

I was filled with passion and determination.
Nothing could put out my fire.
I made hundreds of thousands and drove fine cars.
But I fell, like a falling star.

Now I walk with pride, but I'm shattered inside.
Trying to find my footing, but with every step I slip—this is a horrible trip.

I do believe in me.
I believe that I have a destiny.
Yearning for my twin flame.
Hungering to be financially whole again.

My life is in a constant state of disarray; hopefully, I will admit it to myself one day so that I can remove all doubt and find my way out.

Will any woman love me through my struggles, or am I stuck in this solitary bubble?
Taking responsibility is in my control.
There has to be a reason I keep missing my business goals.

I fell and got back up, but I am still down.
It's time to seek therapy so that I can remove this frown.

I know so much, but even billionaires have a mentor, so it's time for me to find someone to help me center.

I had it all, and I intend to find out: how did I fall?
So that I can once again stand tall.

Time to look deep within.
I know I am a King who deserves to win!

{What Am I Doing Here?}

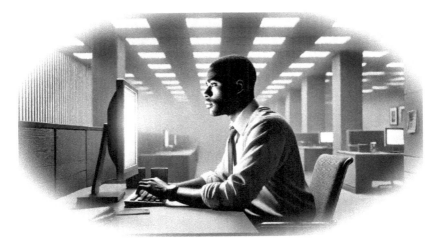

What am I doing here?
A person with so much talent, so much passion,
and so much ambition—trapped,
a prisoner of Corporate Canada.
A job that so many wished they had, but a curse that
I despise!
Why do I compromise?
Hindering my ability to explode, I sit here in this
nightmare and erode.
Day after day, behind this desk, I rot away,
as my creative mind seeks to find the exit sign.

This computer screen is darkening my vision,
my ability to see beyond, my ability to be born—
born into my destiny.
Yes, I was born to be free:
no boss, no chains, no strains.
Wake up when I want to,
go to sleep when I choose to, deal with my own
complaints—no restraints.

Go where no person has gone before, obtaining much more than what the system can give me.
I shall sustain my integrity.

The birds are singing in my ears, "Come, fly."
Ground-bound, I sit down in the master's seat as my talents die.

Hear this true fact:
This corporate job thing is whack.
I shall be my own General, own Captain, own Lieutenant,
My own Commander, only taking orders from my spiritual Director.

"What am I doing here?" is a question I ask no more, for, very soon, I'm walking out the door!

{A Moment Gone}

I wanted to hold you, but I waited too long.
I wanted to tell you I loved you, to make right what was wrong.

How did we get to the point where we threw words of hurt back and forth?
I hurt you, so you hurt me back.
We should have fixed it and gotten back on track.
We should have gone for counseling and stayed consistent. Why weren't we more persistent?

The longer we stayed apart, the more bitterness grew in our hearts, throwing blame back and forth, being extremely mean, like we were quarterbacks on opposing football teams.

The reality is we were both to blame.
We let our pride take over us—what a shame.
At some point, we heard but didn't listen.
Then we listened but refused to understand.
We should have thought the best of each other instead of always thinking negatively, which would have made it easier to forgive.

You meant more to me than the air that I breathe, but how was I to know that your breath would have been your last.
That your life would have ended so fast.
I wanted to hold you, but I waited too long.
I wanted to tell you I loved you, to make right what was wrong.

{The Sun Has Come Out}

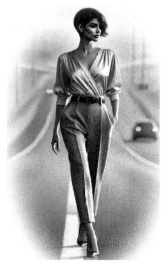

When you left me,
you took a part of me with you.
Left me feeling sad and blue.
How was I supposed to go on?
I didn't think that
I could be strong.
But I want you to
know that I made it over.
The sun has come out again.
My heart has released the pain.
You won't control me anymore.
My soul has been restored.

All those broken promises drove a stake
through my being.
You were the King of spades, and I was the Queen
of hearts.
It doesn't matter any longer because
I've made a brand-new start.

Boy, you did me wrong, and I'm moving on.
I've found my joy.
My emotions are not your toy.

So you can keep your thunderstorms and your rain.
I'm serving you notice that I will love again.
Yes, the sun has come out and the pain is gone.
I want you to know that I'm moving on.

I've found my course; I'm on the right track
Boy, listen up, I'm not coming back!

{You Escalate}

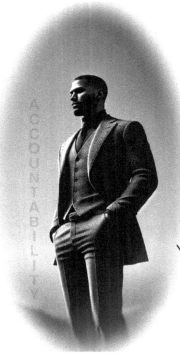

You escalate my joy.
You escalate my pain.
You escalate my love.
You escalate my shame.

You escalate my hormones.
You escalate my anxiety.
You escalate anger.
You escalate my sobriety.

You escalate happiness.
You escalate my sadness.
You escalate my frustration.
You escalate my compassion.

You escalate my fear.
You escalate my despair.
You escalate my dreams.
You escalate my self-esteem.
You escalate my actions.
You escalate my reactions.

I just realized that you didn't do a thing because I am responsible for how I act and react;
for how I allow things to make me feel.
I determine what is true, what is real.

You can try and influence me, but I determine what I accept and reject.
As I pontificate,

it is definitely I, who chose to escalate.

{The Time Has Come}

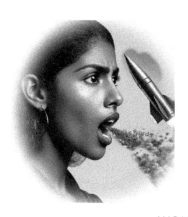

The time has come
for me to confess,
that I will no longer
tolerate the stress.
The stress of communication
that's so caustic.
An unhealthy union, so toxic.
Like a ballistic missile,
your words targeted the
things I confessed to
you in trust, reopening
wounds that took so long to heal.
Once again, turning my heart back to steel.

The time has come to make a decision.
Will I continue to let you suck the life out of my soul,
or will I walk away so I can become whole?
I find myself sinking into a
deep, dark chasm of fury.
Because you've been my prosecutor,
my judge, and my jury.

I am changing course.
I am done accepting this destructive force.
I must love myself enough to believe I deserve more.
Finding the strength to walk through the door.
Straight to therapy is what I need.
To heal the wounds and stop the bleed.
Ending the cycle of choosing wrong.
Today I find my power; I stand strong.

{To Miss You}

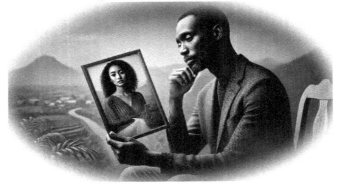

To miss you, baby, is to feel like
I'm missing a part of me.
To miss you, baby, is to stare at your photo endlessly,
amazed by your beauty.
To miss you, baby, is to count the days that you've been away,
wondering when you will come back to stay.

To miss you, baby, is to remember the moments we shared, when you assured me that you cared.
To miss you, baby, is to remember the cold days I held you close to me and your love warmed my body.
To miss you, baby, is to know that we are truly a gift to each other, my true lover.

To miss you, baby, is to miss the best part of me.
You're my harmonic destiny.
To miss you, is longing to kiss you.
To be stuck on you like crazy glue.
To miss you is one of the hardest things
I've ever had to endure.
Come back and be my cure.

{Candy Love}

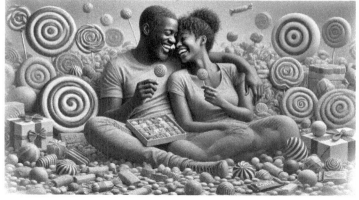

If love were a candy, you'd be too sweet,
If love were a candy, you'd be
the world's greatest treat.

If love were a candy, all others you'd beat.
If love were a candy, you'd be the only kind I eat.

If sweetness were magnetic,
there would not be any left on earth,
For it would have all stuck to you from your birth.

If bees no longer made honey,
what would the world do?
I have the answer: they would all come running to you.

If love were a candy, oh what pleasure divine,
If love were a candy, I hope you'd be all mine.

If love were a candy!

{Loving You Without A Reason}

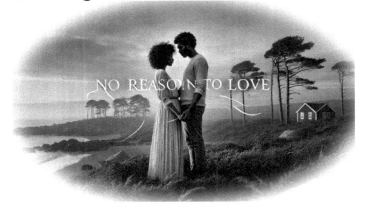

I have no reason for loving you.
I have no reason for wanting to give you the world.
I have no reason for thinking about you with each breath I take.
I have no reason for falling in love with you all those years ago.
I have no reason for letting this love grow.

I have no reason for wanting to keep you smiling all day long.
I have no reason for making you my love song.
The song that gives me joy.
The chorus in my heart.
This love had no reason to start.

Because I had no reason to start,
I have no reason to stop.
Love with no conditions is my mission.

If there are reasons to love you, then there are reasons not to love you.
So, I choose to love without reason in every season.

{When I Love Again}

When I love again, I will love through
the good times and the pain.
When I love again, I will lay my heart out
for her to wrap with care.
When I love again,
I will love void of fear.

I will inhale her.
I will take the deepest breath,
sucking her pheromones
down into the deepest part of me.
When I love again, there will
be no hesitance to give her all of me.
Give everything I am and hope to be.
We will love so freely.

When I love again, honesty will be our way.
Integrity and loyalty will be what I pay
for a love void of conditions.
A love with a singular mission
so that we are walking hand in hand.
She will be my Queen, and I her Superman.
When she slips, I will lift her and help her stand,
when I love again.

I will be with someone who seeks to understand
before she seeks to blame.
She will add to my peace, and I will exalt her name,
giving her all the love languages she desires.
Lifting her higher
and higher as our love stays on fire.

When I love again!

{Sealed, Unsealed, Sealed}

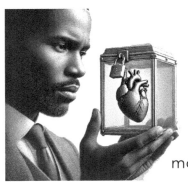

You came and caused me to rip open the seal that enclosed my heart, and you filled it with so much jubilation beyond my imagination. I was energized, beaming from ear to ear, which made me boast. Like the warmth of a monsoon, you held me close.

It was invigorating just to share the same breath with you as our lips locked and our hips knocked. Our bodies intertwined, but the only penetration was our souls dancing in the spiritual realm.

I was in awe, falling deeper in while at the same time soaring higher. With every desire to share a new moment, a new memory with you. You opened my love to a place it had not been in years but then you allowed the fear of a broken heart to bring it all to tears.
I understand but can't pretend that it doesn't hurt. Can't pretend that this burning fire you lit inside of me doesn't want to be put out for fear that the kindle will not reignite as it gets drowned in an ocean of emotions. Back sealed behind a wall of self-sabotage. What could have been? What should have been? What still could be if we set ourselves free of fear, while love is still in the air.

{The Journey Is Over}

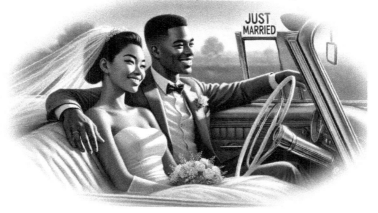

As hard to find as a four-leaf clover,
I've found you, and the journey is over.

A journey filled with highs and lows,
disappointments and failures, laughter and sorrow.
I am so glad that there'll be no searching tomorrow,
because I've found you.

You flew into my life like an eagle flies into the sun.
As soon as you arrived, I knew you were the one.

The vibrations of your voice, your spiritual and mental
state, your astounding beauty assured me it was fate.
Fate that intertwined our destiny not to just to share
our time on earth but our eternity.

You hold me up like the foundation holds a tower.
You help me fulfill my purpose—every moment, every
second, every minute, every hour.

I make mistakes, and you never yell.
Always explaining in a loving way

how I can do better today.
You allow me to lead, and I ask your advice.
We work together lovingly to build this happy life.
I believe the best about you, and you believe the best about me, so we always ask each other for clarification to avoid unnecessary frustrations.

Your desires matter to me, and my desires matter to you, so sometimes we stop and do what the other person wants to do.

We've made a decision not to be upset over something without the other person knowing. Addressing concerns timely and privately when they happen so that our love can keep on growing.

Instead of pointing blame, we stop and evaluate our actions and reactions to see if there is something we could have done better because we believe the other has our best interest at heart.

We apologize for how we made each other feel and we recognize that the discomfort we are experiencing could be because there is some truth to what may have been said, but we swallow our pride and let our joy and love survive.

My shining light, my bright sun,
I am so glad that I have discovered, that the journey is over and a new journey has just begun.